Sirtfood Diet Cookbook

The Essential Guide to Burn Fat Activating Your "Skinny Gene" with 50 Quick and Easy Recipes Ready in 30 Minutes.

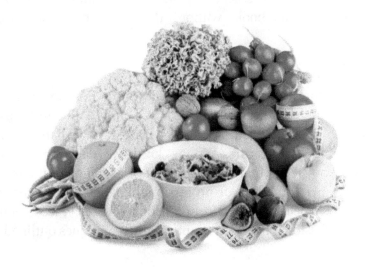

© Copyright 2021 by **Patricia Monroe**

WARNING

The information in this book is for informational purposes only. It is not medical advice or medical opinion and should not be construed as such in any way. Before starting the Sirt diet or taking the foods and/or supplements recommended for this diet, always seek advice from a trusted physician or qualified nutritionist. This is essential to avoid possible side effects. We disclaim any responsibility for any ailments or problems should you decide to follow the Sirt diet or take any foods or supplements associated with this diet.

Table of Contents

CHAPTER 1 - Sirt Diet.. 7

The Benefits..8

What are Sirt foods 8

Allowed foods 9

How the Sirt diet works 10

Solid Meals...11

Contraindications of the Sirt Diet... 12

Green Juice Recipe.. 13

CHAPTER 2 - Foods of the Sirt Diet 15

Tips 19

CHAPTER 3 - Sample Menus 21

CHAPTER 4 - Juices and Smoothies Recipes 25

Red cabbage juice..25

Cucumber and apple juice 26

Green Ginger Juice..28

Coconut milk, kale, turmeric and mint smoothie 29

Smoothie with cherries, banana and mint 30

Spring Green Smoothie... 31

Mango, apple and turmeric smoothie 32

Orange, goji berries and turmeric smoothie 34

Spinach and strawberry smoothie..35

Peaches and raspberries smoothie 36

Avocado and pineapple smoothie...38

Kiwi and banana smoothie 39

Apricots and yogurt smoothie 40

Berry Smoothie... 41

Smoothie with apple and carrot 42

Peach and apricot smoothie..43

Smoothie avocado, mango and orange juice 44

Red fruit smoothie bowl 45

Blackberry and Banana Smoothie... 46

Smoothie bowl with oats and red berries 48

Smoothie bowl banana and cocoa... 50

Mango and banana smoothie bowl 52

CHAPTER 5 - Breakfast Recipes 55

Light Cacao Protein Pudding 55

Ribes Pancakes 56

Cabbage and apple salad 58

Buckwheat and mushroom pancakes 60

Buckwheat Porridge.. 62

CHAPTER 6 - Lunch and Dinner Recipes 65

Scramble Eggs.. 65

Chicken with red onion and black cabbage 67

Chicken and arugula salad 69

Chicken breast baked with walnut and parsley pesto 71

Turkey With Cauliflower Cous 73

Dahl of kale and red onion with buckwheat 75

Baked tofu with harissa 77

Paccheri in miso sauce, broccoli and dried apricots 79

Red quinoa salad.. 81

Quinoa and tuna salad.. 83

Whole wheat penne with broccoli... 86

Quinoa with zucchini and pine nuts 87

Oriental prawns with buckwheat 89

Veggie Burgers 90

Eggplant burgers... 90

Chickpea burger..91

Lentil burger 92

Chapter 7- Gluten-free 93

Braised beef with balsamic vinegar and onions 93

Baked high omelette..96

Mullet fillets with aromatic herbs..98

Pan-fried broccoli...100

Herb soup with chickpeas and speck 102

Basmati rice with chicken and vegetables...104

Ligurian style meatloaf 106

APPENDIX **109**

CHAPTER 1 - Sirt Diet

The Sirtfood Diet is a strict diet that speeds up the metabolism and allows you to lose 3 kg per week: let's see what the Sirt diet is, how it works and what foods are allowed to lose weight fast.

Those who have been trying to lose weight for a long time have surely tried thousands of different diets. Some of them are followed because they are "trendy", but in the end they are not very effective.

New fad diets seem to appear regularly and the Sirtfood diet is one of the latest.

The Sirt diet is on everyone's lips right now and it's being talked about a lot because, unlike most diets, it allows foods like chocolate and red wine, which is good news for foodies who want to lose weight without giving up pleasures.

So let's find out how the Sirt diet works and what are the menus of the diet program.

The Sirt diet is a slimming program that allows you to lose up to 3 kg in a week while staying healthy and fit.

It was created by two British nutritionists, Aidan Goggins and Glen Matten.

The two British nutritionists studied a program according to which a diet based on certain specific foods can promote rapid weight loss.

Unlike others, this slimming program is not only based on a diet of fruits and vegetables, but also offers more freedom in the choice of food, allowing even chocolate.

The Benefits

The Sirt diet is based on the introduction of Sirt foods into our eating regimen, which produce the same beneficial effects as fasting but without the disadvantages.

The creators of this diet claim that following the Sirt diet will lead to rapid weight loss, maintenance of muscle mass and protection from cancer and chronic diseases.

Among the many benefits, in addition to weight loss, there are control of blood sugar levels and improvement of memory; moreover, this diet would be able to clean cells from the accumulation of harmful free radicals.

What are Sirt foods

They are foods particularly rich in special nutrients of vegetable origin and recently discovered, which, stimulated by fasting, activate the genes of thinness.

Lean genes are sirtuins, super regulators of metabolism; these genes influence our mood, our ability to burn fat, and even the mechanisms that regulate longevity.

The sirtuins, however, specialists say, must be activated.

Yes, but how? Normally with exercise and fasting.

The Sirt Diet plan includes a menu that mimics fasting, so as to activate the sirtuins and set the "lean gene" in motion.

Translated with www.DeepL.com/Translator (free version)

Allowed foods

The foods suggested in the Sirt diet, are fresh, wholesome and readily available.

They are not strange or uncommon foods.

Among the others we remember:

- Extra virgin olive oil
- Dark chocolate
- Citrus fruits
- Strawberries
- Apples
- Cabbage
- Celery
- Spinach
- Buckwheat
- Blueberries
- Walnuts
- Soybeans
- Radicchio
- Red onion
- Arugula
- Coffee
- Green tea
- Red wine
- Chili pepper

Then there are tofu, turmeric and medium dates.

In addition, combined with each other or with other foods, they allow you to create very tasty dishes.

How the Sirt diet works

The lean gene diet is not difficult to follow and is divided into two phases.

Phase 1

The first phase has the duration of 7 days and is more restrictive and difficult, especially for the first 3 days.

To be able to lose 3 kg per week as promised by this diet, it is advisable to initially not exceed 1000 calories per day during the first 3 days, drinking 3 green juices based on sirtuin-rich foods and eating only one solid meal of your choice, prepared according to the rules prescribed by the two nutritionists.

From day 4 to day 7, then, you can get up to 1500 calories per day by consuming three green juices and two solid meals consisting of sirtuin-rich foods.

At the end of the seven days, you should have lost, on average, 3.2 pounds.

Phase 2

The second phase, which is the maintenance phase, you'll find it better specified in the book, and it lasts for 14 days.

During this period there are no caloric restrictions but indications on which Sirt foods you need to consume in order to consolidate the weight loss and not run the risk of regaining the kilos lost.

The diet includes specific recipes for those who are vegetarian.

Sirt green juices, recommended in the diet, must be taken in three moments of the day:

- One upon awakening
- One at mid-morning
- One at mid-afternoon.

Phase 1: Typical daily menu

- Breakfast: one Sirt green juice
- Snack: one Sirt green juice
- Lunch: one solid meal, regular or vegan.
- Snack: one Sirt green juice

After the first three days of Phase 1, when the solid meals become two, incorporate a solid dinner as well.

Solid Meals

In general, you can eat foods that are high in protein and low in fat.

Among the meat recipes, you can choose for example Chicken with red onion and kale, Turkey with cauliflower cous cous, (read the recipes below in this article), turkey escalope with capers and parsley.

For fish dishes, sautéed salmon fillet, sautéed king prawns or baked marinated cod are good.

Light and tasty side dish recipes can be prepared with beans, lentils, eggplant cut into wedges and baked, Waldorf salad or red onion salad.

And for dessert, the delicious and healthy strawberries, very high in sirtuins.

Remember, too, that 15-20 g of dark chocolate is allowed every day.

Contraindications of the Sirt Diet

The Sirt diet is not recommended for children and adolescents, underweight, depleted or convalescing persons, and in the presence of nutritional deficiencies or eating disorders.

Moreover, it should be followed only under medical advice and control by pregnant or lactating women, elderly people and menopausal ladies, and in case of diabetes, metabolic diseases, liver and kidney problems, gastrointestinal disorders and chronic diseases.

Green Juice Recipe

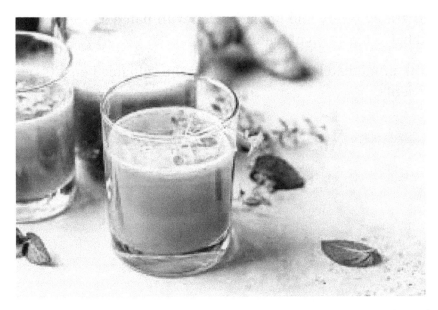

Green juice is an important part of the diet, because it has the ability to cleanse and detoxify, and will be the star in the first week of the Sirt program.

Ingredients

- 75 g of kale
- 30 g of arugula
- 5 g of parsley
- 150 g of green celery with leaves
- 1/2 green apple
- 1/2 lemon juice
- 1/2 teaspoon matcha tea

Preparation

Centrifuge kale, arugula and parsley.

Add grated celery and apple; enrich with half a squeezed lemon and half a teaspoon of matcha tea.

Drink immediately so you don't lose the valuable benefits of the nutrients.

CHAPTER 2 - Foods of the Sirt Diet

RED WINE

The research that originated this diet started right from this drink. The first Sirt "slimming" element discovered, in fact, is resveratrol, present in the skin of black grapes and in red wine. It seems that this nutrient attacks fat cells. In addition, red wine contains piceatannol, which is associated with longevity.

KALE CABBAGE

This is a suitable food for any diet, inexpensive and easy to find. It contains in large quantities two sirtuin-activating nutrients: kaempferol and quercetin, which act synergistically to prevent fat formation.

CACAO

Chocolate yes, but not all of it! It must be dark and contain at least 85% cocoa. Especially useful to appease hunger during the "snack" and the snack.

SARACEN WHEAT

This "pseudo-cereal" is very popular in Japan and is a nutritious and highly satiating food, properties on which this type of nutrition is based.

So yes to buckwheat seeds, flakes and pasta.

CELERY

The nutritive parts of celery, used for thousands of years also as a medicinal plant, are the heart and the leaves: here, in fact, are contained the activators of sirtuins, which are apigenin and luteolin.

An advice: if you can, choose the green one instead of the white one.

THAI CHILI

This food goes to attract metabolism and works on sirtuin due to the presence of luteolin and myricetin. Thai chili, however, is much hotter than regular chili...if you're not used to it, use only half of it and remove the seeds.

MATCHA GREEN TEA

This quality of tea, a key ingredient in the famous green juices, contains the sirtuin activator EGCG. The authors recommend using the Japanese quality.

MEDJOOL DATES

It's true that they are 66% sugar, but they also contain "good" polyphenols that activate sirtuins. So, unlike normal sugars, the nutrients in dates do not increase the amount of glucose in the blood, but their consumption seems instead to be associated with a lower incidence of diabetes and heart disease.

CAPER

The caper plant is widespread in Mediterranean countries and its fruits are very appreciated for their "concentrated taste" capable of reviving even the most anonymous dishes.

Taste aside, capers are also very rich in active-sirtuine nutrients, such as kaempferol and quercitina.

COFFEE

Surprised that coffee is a Sirt food? Here's what Goggins and Matten think: "Contrary to popular opinion that it's harmful, several studies claim that coffee consumption is linked to several health benefits." According to the creators of the diet, in fact, coffee would protect the liver and defend the body from diabetes, some cancers and neurodegenerative diseases.

EXTRA VIRGIN OLIVE OIL

Good and healthy, extra virgin olive oil, obtained from the first pressing of olives, is a perfect condiment, delicious on vegetables as well as on bread!

Rich in polyphenols, fatty acids "good" and vitamin E, is a friend of the heart and youth, thanks to its antioxidant properties.

ARUGULA

Arugula is a vegetable rich in nutrients that activate the metabolism, such as quercitina and kaempferol. Its peppery and strong flavor can embellish many recipes, especially when accompanied by olive oil.

A curiosity: it was cultivated for the first time in ancient Rome, where it seems it was very appreciated for its aphrodisiac properties...

PARSLEY

It is a basic ingredient to enrich practically any dish and a lot of sauces. It has a fresh flavor, and is used to relieve itching and toothache.

The Sirt diet especially values it because it is one of the foods with the highest concentration of apigenin, a sirtuin activator.

RED CHICORY

It is famous in the form of radicchio and can be consumed in the diet, in large quantities, either alone or accompanied by other Sirt foods.

SOY

In addition to its beneficial properties, associated with the activating action of daidzein and formononetin, soy has an unmistakable flavor that makes every dish tasty.

Soy sauce, soy yogurt and miso, a traditional Japanese dish based on soybeans fermented with salt, are good. To prepare Sirt recipes, the most suitable qualities are red miso and brown miso.

RED ONION

Tasty and rich in quercitina, which activates the metabolism. It is important to peel it and eat it raw to keep the nutrients active and act better on sirtuins.

STRAWBERRIES

They have low sugar, are delicious and are also slimming because they are the main source of fisetina, a sirtuin activator.

In addition, Goggins and Matten write that: "scientists have found that if we add strawberries to simple sugars, this causes a reduction in the demand for insulin, and thus transforms food into a sustained energy-releasing machine."

NUTS

They are high in fat and very caloric, yet, according to Sirt nutritionists, this food debunks clichés, as it actually promotes weight loss while also fighting metabolic diseases. In addition, nuts contain a lot of minerals useful to the body such as magnesium, zinc, copper, calcium and iron.

Tips

Chocolate

Choose dark chocolate with 85% cocoa, rich in antioxidants, has a low glycemic index.

Green Tea

Known because it is so good for our body, green tea contributes to fat loss, preserving muscles. Choose the Matcha variety and drink it with the addition of a little lemon juice, which increases the absorption of sirtuin activating nutrients.

Chilli

To spice up your dishes, use Bird's Eye (also called Thai) chili peppers, which are very rich in sirtuin.

You can use it at least three times a week.

Warning!

Compared to normal hot peppers, Bird's Eye is much hotter; to get used to it, at the beginning, use only half of the amount indicated in the recipe, eliminating the seeds, which are very hot.

Coffee

You can drink 3-4 cups a day being careful not to exaggerate with sugar and avoiding the addition of milk.

CHAPTER 3 - Sample Menus

But let's get into the nitty-gritty of this eating style and see an example of the food program, listing the weekly menu. We will start with the green juice, listing daily what to eat between breakfast, lunch and dinner.

It's called the red wine and chocolate diet, but wine is banned in week 1 (thereafter you can consume 2-3 glasses per week). Chocolate remains for the first few days in the form of a snack or treat.

Monday

- Breakfast: water + tea or espresso + 1 cup of green juice;
- Lunch: green juice (3 cups total in a day);
- Snack: one square of dark chocolate;
- Dinner: buckwheat pasta + vegetables and chicken.
- After dinner: one square of dark chocolate.

Tuesday

- Breakfast: water + tea or espresso + 1 cup of green juice (3 times a day),
- Lunch: 2 green juices before dinner;
- Snack: a square of dark chocolate;
- Dinner: couscous with vegetables + chicken or shrimp.
- After dinner: a square of dark chocolate.

Wednesday

- Breakfast: water + tea or espresso + 1 cup of green juice (3 times a day),
- Lunch: 2 green juices before dinner;
- Snack: a square of dark chocolate;
- Dinner: plenty of vegetables + chicken or fish;
- Post dinner: a square of dark chocolate.

Thursday

- Breakfast: water + tea or espresso + 1 cup of green juice (2 times a day),
- Lunch: Sirt Muesli;
- Snack: one green juice before dinner;
- Dinner: vegetable soup with beans.

Friday

- Breakfast: water + tea or espresso + 1 cup of green juice (2 times a day);
- Lunch: buckwheat salad with vegetables;
- Snack: one green juice before dinner;
- Dinner: grilled fish or meat + side of vegetables and baked potatoes.

Saturday

- Breakfast: a bowl of that delicious Sirt Muesli + 1 cup of green juice
- Lunch: Sirtfood omelette with bacon;
- Snack: 1 cup of green juice;
- Dinner: chicken with walnuts and parsley + a red onion + tomato salad.

Sunday

-   Breakfast: water + tea or espresso + 1 cup of green juice (2 times a day);
-   Lunch: Sirt salad + grilled fish or chicken;
-   Snack: 1 cup of green juice;
-   Dinner: fish or meat cooked with a dash of red wine + plenty of salad and vegetables.

Patricia Monroe

CHAPTER 4 - Juices and Smoothies Recipes

Red cabbage juice

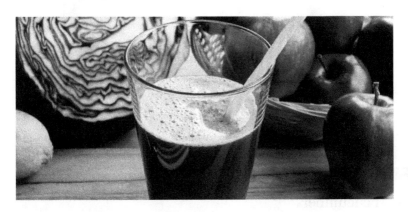

Ingredients for 2 persons:

- 200 g of red cabbage
- 1 fennel
- 2 oranges
- 10 g of cleaned ginger

Preparation:

Clean the ingredients, peel the oranges, removing the white skin, then extract the juice from the cabbage, fennel, oranges and ginger.

Cucumber and apple juice

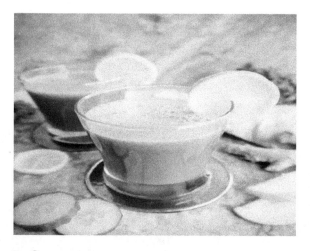

Ingredients for 2 persons:

- 1 cucumber
- 2 yellow apples
- 30 grams of lemon
- 4 mint leaves
- 3 basil leaves

Preparation:

Wash the fruits and vegetables well.

Peel the cucumber and cut it into pieces if necessary. The skin can also be left on, but it gives the juice a more bitter taste.

Remove the stems from the apples and cut them into wedges.

Remove the zest from the lemon and cut it into two pieces. The lemon can be used with the peel only if edible. The lemon zest gives the juice a more bitter flavor.

Insert the fine mesh filter into the extractor of the blender.

Close the airtight spout.

Start the extractor and add the ingredients alternately, leaving the mint and basil leaves for last.

Decorate the juice with a few remaining mint leaves.

Green Ginger Juice

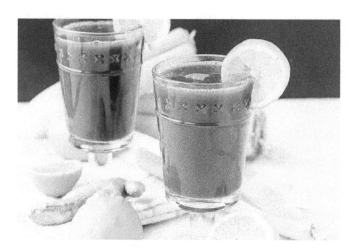

Ingredients for 2 persons:

-   120 ml of water
-   300 g of cucumber (1 cucumber)
-   80 g celery (½ stalk)
-   375 g apples (2 medium apples), seeded and cut in half
-   60 g of kale
-   5 g fresh ginger root, peel off

Preparation:

Place all ingredients inside the blender jug in the order listed and close the lid. Select speed 1. Start the appliance and slowly increase to full speed.

Blend for 30-45 seconds, using the press to push the ingredients toward the blades. If using a blender with programs, select the Smoothie program button and wait for the programmed cycle to complete. Strain using a vegetable milk filter bag. Store in the refrigerator. Use within 2 days.

Coconut milk, kale, turmeric and mint smoothie

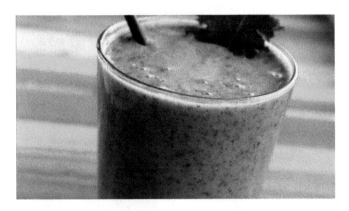

Ingredients for 2 persons:

- 6 leaves of black cabbage, without central rib
- 50 gr of rocket
- 200 ml of coconut milk
- Two pieces of fresh turmeric root
- One citron
- 4 or 5 peppermint leaves

Preparation:

First, wash the kale leaves and arugula and dry well;

Remove the central rib from the kale leaves and chop them into pieces in a blender with 100 ml of coconut milk;

Now add the arugula, mint and another 100 ml of coconut milk and blend;

Squeeze the citron, cut the turmeric root into small pieces and pour it into the blender together with the citron juice for 30 seconds; If it turns out not very liquid, add more coconut milk until desired consistency. Your smoothie is ready to enjoy!

Smoothie with cherries, banana and mint

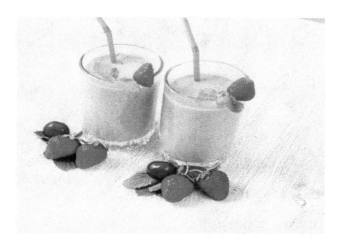

Ingredients for 2 persons:

- 1 ripe banana
- 3 washed and dried Mint leaves
- 1 sprig of Parsley washed and dried (optional)
- Rice Milk
- 1 cup of Pitted Cherries

Preparation:

Take a ripe banana, peel it and chop it coarsely, then wash and dry the parsley and mint; Wash and stone the cherries, which you will keep aside;

Add the banana, mint and parsley to the blender, then pour in the rice milk until you get the desired consistency, about 1 cup. If you don't have this drink you can substitute it with water or another vegetable milk;

Blend all the ingredients for about a minute, then add the cherries and blend again for another minute; Pour into glass and drink. You can also prepare a small plate with some cherries to snack on along with the smoothie.

Spring Green Smoothie

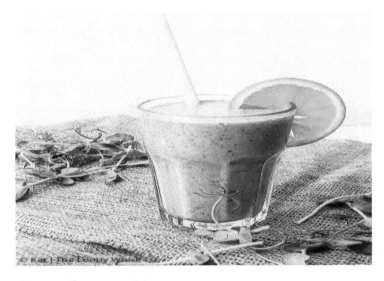

Ingredients for 1 persons:

- 1 Kiwi Rice milk
- 1 Ripe Banana
- 1 large lettuce leaf

Preparation:

Take a ripe banana, peel it and cut it into coarse prices;

Take a kiwi, peel it and cut it into small pieces as well;

Wash and chop a large lettuce leaf;

At this point add the rice milk until you get the desired consistency, about 4 tablespoons. If you don't have this drink you can replace the rice milk with water;

If you have guests, decorate with a mint leaf and some fresh kiwi slices before serving.

Mango, apple and turmeric smoothie

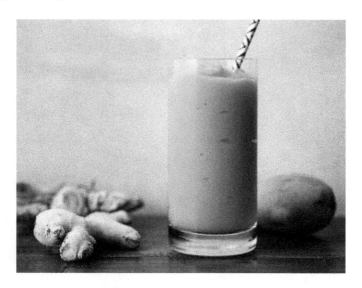

Ingredients for 2 persons:

- 400 g of mango
- 300 g of green apple
- 1 teaspoon turmeric
- 1 teaspoon of honey
- the zest of 1 lime
- 10 leaves of oregano
- 2-3 cm of fresh ginger
- 250 ml of water

Preparation:

To make the mango, green apple and turmeric smoothes, first we wash the mango, lime, apple and oregano. We need to clean all the ingredients well and avoid the presence of impurities.

Then we peel the ripe mango and apple and cut the pulp of both into small pieces.

We take the blender, we pour the pieces of fruit just obtained, the ginger previously peeled and cut into small pieces, the lime zest, the juice of the lime and all other ingredients.

Blend everything after adding about 250 ml of water into the glass. The liquid should have a smooth and uniform consistency. The ingredients should blend together as well as possible.

Orange, goji berries and turmeric smoothie

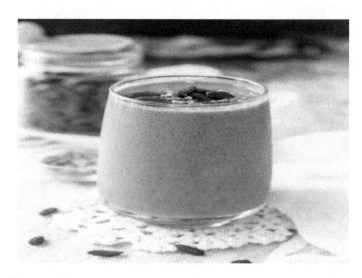

Ingredients for 2 persons:

- 2 oranges
- Half a tablespoon of turmeric powder
- Half a tablespoon of grated ginger
- 3 tablespoons of goji berries
- About half a cup of water

Preparation:

After squeezing the oranges, we blend all the ingredients until we get a smooth consistency. We can also add some ice cubes for a cooler drink.

To make the result even more spectacular, we can decorate the glass with half an orange slice. It is recommended to drink this smoothie in the morning to enjoy a day full of energy.

Spinach and strawberry smoothie

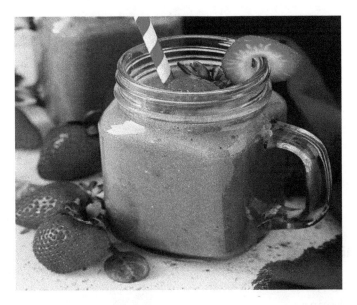

Ingredients for 4 persons:

- 1 cup fresh strawberries
- 1 banana
- 1 cup orange juice
- 1 cup almond milk, unsweetened
- 500gr fresh baby spinach
- 1 cup of ice
- 8 to 16 packets of sugar to achieve desired level of sweetness

Preparation:

Place all ingredients in a kitchen mixer.

Turn the blender on high speed until smooth.

*This smoothie has 90 calories and 15 grams of sugar per serving.

Peaches and raspberries smoothie

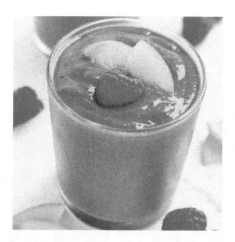

Ingredients for 2 persons:

- 125 g of raspberries
- 1 banana
- 1 peach
- 1 pot of white yogurt
- 100 ml of milk
- 2 tablespoons of honey

To decorate

- banana slices
- peach slices
- raspberries
- shelled walnuts

Preparation:

First we cut up the banana, peach and raspberries and pour everything into the glass of the mixer.

Add the pot of yogurt, milk and two tablespoons of honey.

We blend everything, then we transfer our smoothie in a cup.

Decorate with banana slices, peach slices and raspberries.

Add some shelled walnuts and possibly some poppy seeds and at this point we can enjoy our smoothie.

Avocado and pineapple smoothie

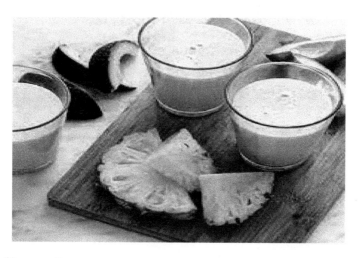

Ingredients for 2 persons:

- 100 g pineapple pieces
- 100 g avocado pulp
- 2 tablespoons of honey
- 300 ml of almond milk
- raspberries to decorate

Preparation:

We start by cutting the pineapple and avocado pulp into pieces, after which we pour them into the mixer glass along with two tablespoons of honey.

We add the almond milk and blend everything.

We pour our smoothie in two glasses and decorate with raspberries: now the smoothie is ready to be enjoyed.

Kiwi and banana smoothie

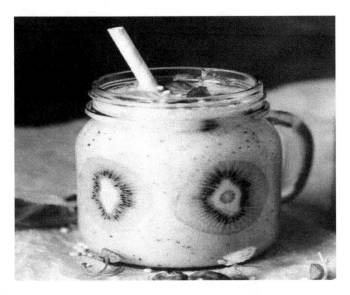

Ingredients for 2 persons:

- 3 kiwi
- 1 banana
- 100 ml of milk

Preparation:

First let's peel the kiwis; we used the Golden variety, but other varieties are also fine, the important thing is that the fruit is ripe. Cut them into slices and then into smaller pieces.

We peel and cut into rounds a banana and transfer everything into a mixer.

Blend until the fruit is reduced to a creamy puree, then pour in the milk.

Blend for a few more moments to blend and pour into glasses, decorate them with kiwi slices and enjoy our delicious kiwi and banana smoothie.

Apricots and yogurt smoothie

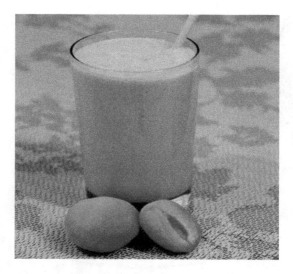

Ingredients for 1 persons:

- 6 apricots
- 125 ml of white yogurt
- 2 tablespoons of brown sugar

Preparation:

To prepare this drink, we choose ripe apricots, wash them, cut them in half and then into smaller pieces, removing the stone.

Blend everything until reduced to a puree.

We join the white yogurt and two tablespoons of brown sugar. If the apricots were not sweet enough, we can increase the dose of sugar: taste and adjust according to our tastes.

Blend again to make the mixture homogeneous and finally transfer it into a glass that we can garnish with a tuft of fresh mint.

Berry Smoothie

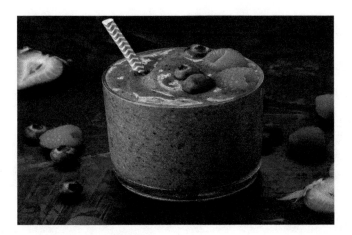

Ingredients for 4 persons:

- 120 g of blueberries
- 120 ml of sugar syrup
- 140 g of strawberries
- 6 tablespoons of white yogurt
- 10 ice cubes

Preparation:

Wash the berries well under running water and place them in a blender along with the sugar syrup and ice.

Blend everything at moderate speed until you have obtained a fairly dense mixture.

As an alternative to the sugar syrup, you can dissolve 2 teaspoons of caster sugar in two cups of water and pour them into the blender before starting it.

Smoothie with apple and carrot

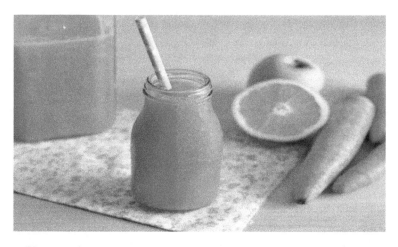

Ingredients for 4 persons:

- 4 medium apples (better if green)
- 300 g of carrots
- 2 stalks of celery
- 2 lemons

Preparation:

Peel the carrots with a knife or potato peeler and wash them thoroughly.

Cut them into very small pieces before putting them in the blender to prevent damage. Peel the apples as well and cut them into small pieces.

Do the same with the celery stalks, taking care to remove the filaments with a small knife. In a glass, squeeze the juice of 2 lemons.

Then put all the ingredients in the blender and start it at medium speed. The smoothie is ready in seconds!

Serve with a slice of lemon and a few mint leaves.

Peach and apricot smoothie

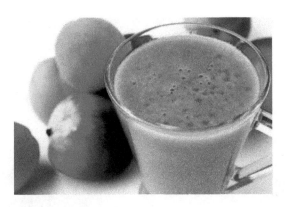

Ingredients for 4 persons:

- 8 ripe apricots
- 5 peaches
- 300 g of strawberries
- 2 spoons of honey
- 1 lemon
- 1 pot of fruit yogurt (optional)

Preparation:

Start by washing all the fruit well and if necessary leave it in a salad bowl with water for about half an hour.

After that you can cut the peaches and apricots into pieces not too small by removing all the stones. Squeeze the lemon in a glass or directly in the blender and add the pot of yogurt.

After cutting the strawberries as well, you can add them to the blender along with the other fruit and honey. Blend everything until the ingredients are completely blended.

It will only take a few seconds and the smoothie will be ready to drink. Since it is very thick you can use a teaspoon as well.

Smoothie avocado, mango and orange juice

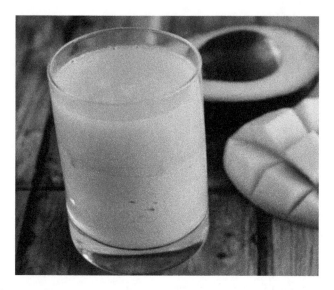

Ingredients for 2 persons:

- 1 avocado
- 1 mango
- the juice of 2 oranges
- 2 teaspoons of goji berries

Preparation:

Let's start preparing the fruit, washing it thoroughly and removing the skin: cut the avocado and mango into cubes, transfer them into the pitcher of a blender, squeeze the juice of the 2 oranges and add it to the fruit. Operate at maximum speed and turn off when the smoothie has taken on a full-bodied consistency.

If we don't have a food processor, we can also use an immersion blender that chops the fruits in a similar way.

Pour it into a pitcher or directly into cocktail glasses, add the goji berries and decorate with an orange slice.

Red fruit smoothie bowl

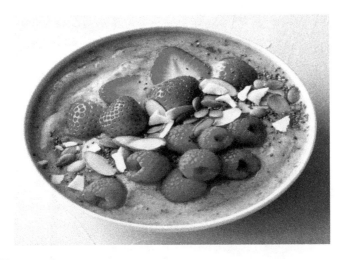

Ingredients for 1 persons:

- 50 g of strawberries
- 50 g of raspberries
- 30 g of blueberries
- 1 pot of Greek yogurt
- grated coconut
- oat flakes

Preparation:

Let's take the strawberries, raspberries and blueberries and wash them.

Then, we put the ingredients inside a blender and start blending.

We add a jar of Greek yogurt in the mixer.

Let's pour the blended red berries with yogurt inside a bowl.

Finally, we can decorate the surface of the smoothie bowl as desired with chopped strawberries, blueberries, raspberries, some oatmeal and grated coconut.

Blackberry and Banana Smoothie

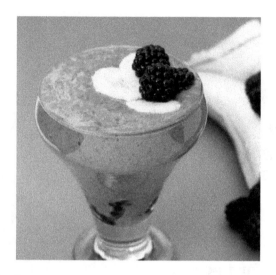

Ingredients for 4 persons:

- 300 g of blackberries
- 2 bananas
- 4 spoons of milk ice cream
- 125 g of white yogurt
- 10 ice cubes

Preparation:

To prepare the blackberry and banana smoothie, we must first thoroughly wash the fresh blackberries under running water and place them inside the pitcher of a blender.

After that, we peel the bananas and cut them into small pieces, then we put them in the mixer. To make the smoothie naturally sweet without adding sugar, we recommend choosing very ripe bananas, but not too dark.

We start blending to obtain a homogeneous puree, then we add the milk ice cream, the white yogurt and, finally, the ice cubes.

We continue blending at maximum power for about a minute but intermittently so as not to overheat the blades, until we get a smooth and perfectly creamy smoothie.

Now that the blackberry and banana smoothie is ready, we just have to serve it to our guests in glass glasses. We can eventually add 1 or 2 whole ice cubes and decorate everything with a few leaves of fresh mint.

Smoothie bowl with oats and red berries

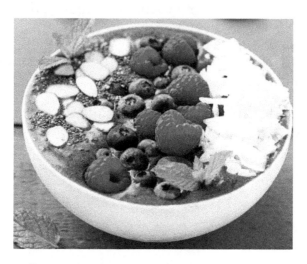

Ingredients for 4 persons:

- 500 of oat milk
- 5 tablespoons of oatmeal
- 4 cups of red fruits
- 2 ripe bananas
- almonds
- chia seeds
- berries for garnish

Preparation:

To prepare the smoothie bowl with oats and red berries, we must first peel the bananas, cut them into slices and place them inside a food bag along with the red berries.

We place the bag inside the freezer and let the fruit freeze overnight.

In a bowl pour 100 ml of oat milk, add the oatmeal and cover the bowl with plastic wrap. Let's place it in the refrigerator and let it rest overnight.

In the morning, pour the soaked oatmeal into a blender, add the remaining oat milk and frozen fruit. We blend everything on maximum power for a few seconds, until we get a smooth and creamy smoothie.

The smoothie bowl with oats and red berries is ready to be garnished on top with the topping of your choice.

Smoothie bowl banana and cocoa

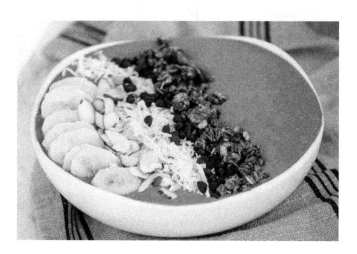

Ingredients for 4 persons:

- 4 bananas
- 340 g of Greek yogurt
- drops of dark chocolate
- 4 teaspoons of bitter cocoa
- 2 teaspoons of wildflower honey
- chopped pistachios
- muesli
- goji berries

Preparation:

To prepare the chocolate and banana smoothie bowl, we must first peel the bananas and cut them into slices. We can possibly freeze them in the freezer for 5-6 hours, or use them at room temperature.

We put the banana slices in a blender and add the remaining ingredients: Greek yogurt, honey and sifted cocoa. Blend everything on maximum power for a few seconds, until you get a thick and creamy smoothie.

Pour the smoothie into 4 glass bowls or cups and level the surface. Now we just have to garnish it with the ingredients chosen for the topping: let's distribute in an orderly manner the goji berries, the dark chocolate chips, the pistachio grains and, finally, the muesli.

The ingredients for the topping can be chosen according to your taste, preferring oil seeds, fresh and dried fruit. Coconut flakes, almonds or toasted hazelnuts are excellent.

We recommend serving the chocolate and banana smoothie bowl immediately.

Mango and banana smoothie bowl

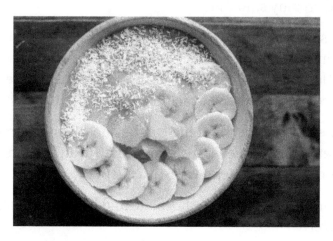

Ingredients for 4 persons:

- 5 Banana
- 4 mango
- 4 pots of Greek yogurt
- sweet almonds
- oatmeal mignon

Preparation:

To prepare the mango and banana smoothie, we must first peel 4 bananas, cut them into small pieces and place them inside the pitcher of a blender.

Having done this, we proceed by cleaning the mangoes and removing the seed present in the center. With the help of a knife, remove the ripe pulp and place it in the blender.

Add the Greek yogurt (or vegetable soy yogurt) and blend at maximum power for a few moments, until you get a thick and creamy smoothie.

We pour the smoothie inside four bowls and proceed with the decoration. Cut the remaining banana into slices and distribute them on the surface of the smoothie. We complete it with the sweet almonds, pumpkin seeds and oatmeal.

The mango-banana smoothie bowl is now ready: we can enjoy it immediately or put it in the fridge for about 30 minutes and serve it cold.

CHAPTER 5 - Breakfast Recipes

Light Cacao Protein Pudding

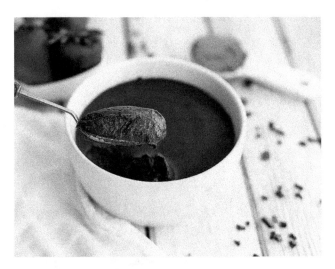

Ingredients for 1 persons:

- 100 gr Albumen
- 100 ml Water
- Bitter cocoa powder (2 level teaspoons)
- 1 teaspoon Honey

Preparation:

1. Pour the water and egg whites into a small saucepan and cook over medium heat. When it starts to boil, leave the flame on for a couple more minutes and then signs.
2. Transfer the mixture to a tall, narrow container, then add the cocoa and honey.
3. Blend everything with a blender, transfer the mixture to a glass and let it cool. It will thicken over time and take on the consistency of a real pudding.

Ribes Pancakes

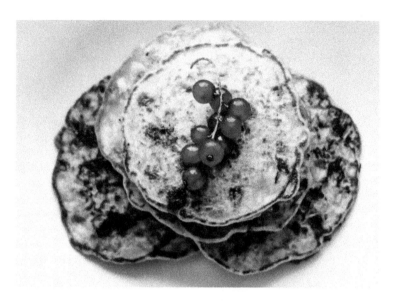

Ingredients for 4 persons:

- Cassis sauce
- 300 g of blackcurrants
- 1 vanilla pod
- 70 g of fine raw cane sugar
- 150 ml of blackcurrant nectar
- 3 El Cassis, (blackcurrant liqueur)
- 1 tablespoon custard powder
- Pancakes
- 25 g butter
- 2 eggs, (class M)
- 200 ml buttermilk
- 40 g of fine raw cane sugar
- 150 g of flour
- 1 tablespoon baking powder

- salt
- 300 g of redcurrants
- 25 g amaretti cookies (Italian almond cookies)
- 5 tablespoons butter and oil
- 2 tablespoons of powdered sugar
- 4 scoops of strawberry ice cream

Preparation:

Blackcurrant with a fork from the cob strips. Cut the vanilla pod lengthwise and scrape out the pith. Caramelise the sugar in a pan until golden brown, stirring until the sugar begins to melt in one place. Deglaze with the nectar, add the vanilla bean and the mark. Add the berries, bring to a boil and cook gently for 5 minutes over medium heat, pass through a fine sieve, bring to a boil again. Stir in cassis and pudding powder until smooth, stir into boiling mixture, boil again, fill into a bowl and let cool.

Melt the butter over medium heat. Stir in eggs, buttermilk and sugar with a whisk. Stir in butter. Stir in the flour, baking powder and a pinch of salt and mix well. Allow dough to puff up at room temperature for 15 minutes.

Red currant strips from the cob. Put the macaroons in a freezer bag and crush them finely. Mix the dough again. Heat 1 of butter and oil in a non-stick skillet (28 cm Ø). Pour the batter into the pan for 4 pancakes (about 8 cm each). Scatter some currants and macaroon crumbs on top. Cook over medium heat for 2-3 minutes until golden brown on each side. Finished pancakes in 120 degree oven (gas 1, circulating air not recommended) keep warm on a baking sheet covered with baking paper. In this way cook in 4-5 servings of 16-20 pancakes. Dust the pancakes with powdered sugar and serve with the sauce and strawberry ice cream.

Cabbage and apple salad

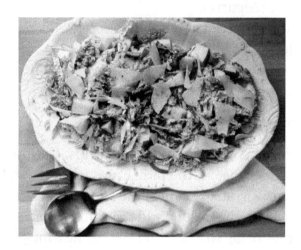

Ingredients for 4 persons:

- 4 tbsp white vinegar
- 26 g whole cane sugar
- 2 tablespoons seed or olive oil
- 4 tablespoons water
- 4 tablespoons mayonnaise
- 2 g paprika
- ¼ cabbage
- 4 spring onions
- 1 green apples
- 1 pinch salt

Preparation:

Place the vinegar, whole grain brown sugar, oil and water in a small saucepan. Cook for 4 minutes over medium heat. Remove from heat. Add mayonnaise and paprika. Season with salt and pepper. Stir well.

Prepare the cabbage and spring onions by cutting them very finely and transferring them to a salad bowl. Peel the apples, remove the core, slice and add to the salad bowl. Pour in the vinaigrette and mix well. Adjust seasoning.

Cover with plastic wrap and refrigerate at least 1 hour before serving.

Buckwheat and mushroom pancakes

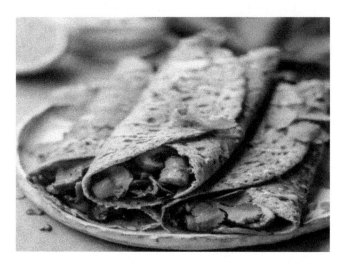

Ingredients for 2 persons:

- 200 g of buckwheat
- 1 package of dried porcini mushrooms
- 1 shallot
- 1 egg
- 3 tablespoons of breadcrumbs
- 3 tablespoons of parmesan cheese
- seed oil
- salt and pepper

Preparation:

Wash the buckwheat with plenty of water, drain it and in the meantime bring the water to a boil (twice the volume of millet, so for 200 gr of buckwheat -> 400 ml of water).

Cook the buckwheat for about 20 minutes and let it rest for another 10 minutes. Meanwhile, soak the mushrooms in a bowl and then rinse them.

In a frying pan, brown the shallot and the mushrooms, squeezed and chopped. Add everything to the buckwheat and let it cool.

Pour the mixture into a bowl, add the beaten egg, 3 tablespoons of breadcrumbs, the other 3 tablespoons of Parmesan cheese, salt and pepper. Bread the fritters and fry them.

Buckwheat Porridge

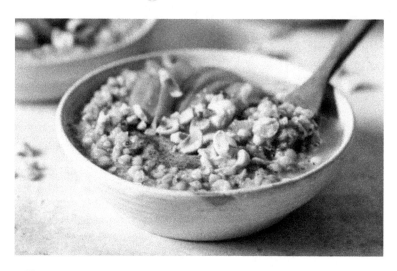

Ingredients for 4 persons:

- 90 g of buckwheat
- 15 g of bitter cocoa
- 130 g of almond milk
- 130 g of water
- 30 g maple syrup
- 40 g pecans
- ½ teaspoon cinnamon
- 1 pinch of vanilla powder
- 1 pinch of chili pepper

Preparation:

Pour the buckwheat, water, almond milk, maple syrup, sifted cocoa, vanilla, cinnamon and chili pepper into a small saucepan, stirring well. Place on the stove, bring to a boil and lower the heat, then cover with a lid. Cook for about 18 minutes, stirring occasionally.

Once all the liquid has been absorbed and the buckwheat is cooked, turn off the flame and let it rest for 10 minutes with the lid on. Serve the oatmeal by pouring it into cups and decorating with the pecans coarsely chopped with a knife.

Patricia Monroe

CHAPTER 6 - Lunch and Dinner Recipes

Scramble Eggs

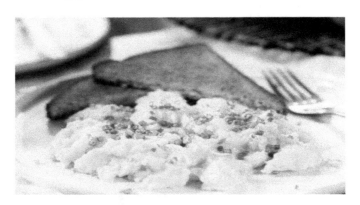

Ingredients for 2 persons:

- 2 Eggs
- 1 tablespoon of Butter
- 6 slices of Bacon
- enough Extra Virgin Olive Oil

Preparation:

1. Start by preparing the eggs. Crack a couple into a bowl, season with salt and pepper. If desired, break up some coarse salt and peppercorns in a mortar for a more intense aroma.
2. Lightly beat the eggs with a fork. Meanwhile, melt a knob of butter in a non-stick frying pan. Cook the bacon slices for a few minutes on each side. They should be golden brown and crispy (not burnt!). Set them aside on a plate.

3. Pour the lightly beaten eggs into the pan and, using a spatula, continue to lift them up on different sides. They should firm up but still remain soft.

Chicken with red onion and black cabbage

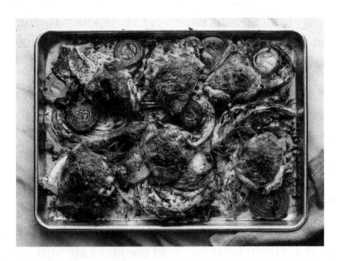

Ingredients for 2 persons:

- 120 g of chicken breast
- 130 g of tomatoes
- 1 hot pepper
- 1 tablespoon capers
- 5 g of parsley
- lemon juice
- 2 tbsp. Extra virgin olive oil
- 2 teaspoons of turmeric
- 50 g of cabbage
- 20 g of red onion
- 1 teaspoon of fresh ginger
- 50 g buckwheat

Preparation:

Marinate chicken breast for 10 minutes with 1/4 lemon juice, 1 tablespoon extra-virgin olive oil and 1 teaspoon turmeric powder.

Cut 130 g tomatoes into small pieces, remove the insides, season with chili, 1 tablespoon capers, 1 teaspoon turmeric and 1 teaspoon extra virgin olive oil, 1/4 teaspoon lemon juice and 5 g chopped parsley.

Fry the chicken breast, drained from the marinade, over high heat for one minute on each side, then place it in the oven for about 10 minutes at 220°C.

Let it rest covered with aluminium foil.

Steam the chopped kale for 5 minutes.

Sauté one red onion, one teaspoon grated fresh ginger and one teaspoon extra virgin olive oil; add cooked kale and cook for one minute on the stove.

Boil buckwheat with a teaspoon of turmeric, drain and serve with chicken, tomatoes and shredded cabbage.

Chicken and arugula salad

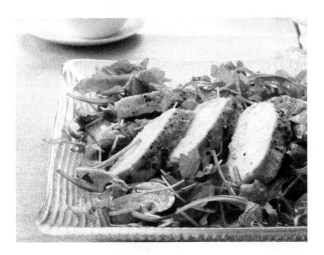

Ingredients for 4 persons:

- 800 g of chicken breast in 4 rather thick slices
- 120 g of rocket
- 150 g of cherry tomatoes
- 2 spoons of pine nuts
- EVO oil
- Salt and pepper

Preparation:

Toast the pine nuts for a minute in a non-stick skillet over low heat. Sauté them continuously because they burn very easily. Set them aside. Wash and dry the arugula in a salad spinner. Put it in a bowl and dress it with a drizzle of oil and a pinch of salt.

Wash the cherry tomatoes, dry them, cut them in half and pour them into another bowl. Dress them with a drizzle of oil and a pinch of salt and pepper. Put a non-stick frying pan on the stove and bring it to heat. Pour in a couple of tablespoons of oil and swirl it around so that it is evenly distributed.

Place the slices of chicken breast in the hot pan and cook them for three minutes, moving them from time to time so that they do not stick and do not burn. Turn the slices of meat, season with salt and pepper and cook for another two minutes. At the end, the chicken breast should be well cooked, even on the inside. Transfer the chicken breast slices to a cutting board and cut them into strips.

On each plate create a bed with the rughetta and sprinkle with pine nuts. Add the cherry tomatoes and place the chicken breast pieces in the center.

Chicken breast baked with walnut and parsley pesto

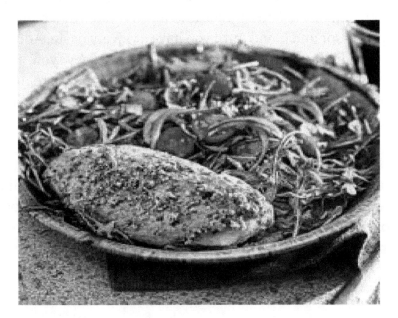

Ingredients for 2 persons:

- 15g parsley,
- 15g of walnuts,
- 15g parmesan cheese,
- 1 tablespoon extra virgin olive oil
- juice of 1/2 lemon
- 50ml water,
- 150g chicken breast without skin
- 20g red onions,
- 1 teaspoon of red wine vinegar,
- 35g rocket,
- 100g cherry tomatoes,
- 1 teaspoon balsamic vinegar.

Preparation:

To make the pesto, place the parsley, walnuts, Parmesan cheese, olive oil, half of the lemon juice and a little water in a blender or food processor and blend until you have a velvety paste. Add more water gradually until you have the consistency you prefer. Marinate the chicken breast in 1 tablespoon of the pesto and the remaining lemon juice in the refrigerator for 30 minutes, longer if possible. Preheat the oven to 200°.

Heat an ovenproof skillet over medium-high heat. Fry the chicken in its marinade for 1 minute on each side, then transfer the pan to the oven and bake for 8 minutes or until cooked through. Marinate the onions in the red wine vinegar for 5-10 minutes. Strain off the liquid.

When the chicken is cooked, remove it from the oven, pour another spoonful of pesto over it and let the heat of the chicken melt it. Cover with aluminium foil and let stand 5 minutes before serving. Stir in arugula, tomatoes and onions and drizzle with balsamic vinegar. Serve with the chicken, drizzling the remaining pesto over the top.

Turkey With Cauliflower Cous

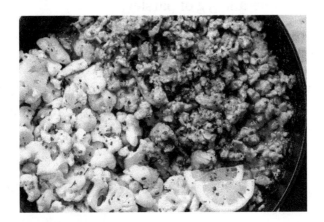

Ingredients for 2 persons:

- 150 g of turkey
- 150 g of cauliflower
- 40 g of red onion
- 1 teaspoon fresh ginger
- 1 pepper
- 1 garlic clove
- 3 tablespoons of extra virgin olive oil
- 2 teaspoons of turmeric
- 30 g of sun-dried tomatoes
- 10 g of parsley
- dried sage
- 1 tablespoon capers
- 1/4 of fresh lemon juice

Preparation:

Blend the raw cauliflower florets and then cook them in a teaspoon of evo oil, the garlic, red onion, chilli, ginger and a teaspoon of turmeric.

Let it season for a minute, then add, with the heat off, the chopped sun-dried tomatoes and 5 g of parsley.

Season the turkey slice with a teaspoon of evo oil, the dried sage and cook it in another teaspoon of evo oil.

When ready, season with one tablespoon capers, 1/4 teaspoon lemon juice, 5 g parsley, one tablespoon water and add the cauliflower.

Dahl of kale and red onion with buckwheat

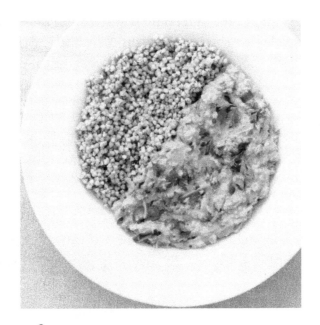

Ingredients for 1 persons:

- 1 teaspoon of extra virgin olive oil
- 1 teaspoon of mustard seeds
- 40g red onion, finely chopped
- 1 garlic clove, finely chopped
- 1 teaspoon fresh ginger, finely chopped
- 1 Bird's Eye chili pepper, finely chopped
- 1 teaspoon sweet (or, if you prefer, medium or hot) curry powder
- 2 teaspoons turmeric powder
- 300ml vegetable stock or water
- 40g red lentils, rinsed
- 50g kale, chopped
- 50ml canned coconut milk
- 50g buckwheat

Preparation:

Heat the oil in a medium saucepan over medium heat and add the mustard seeds. When they begin to crackle, add the onion, garlic, ginger, and chili. Cook for about 10 minutes, until everything is wilted.

Add the curry powder and 1 teaspoon of turmeric, and cook the spices for a couple of minutes. Pour in the broth and bring to a boil. Add the lentils and cook for another 25-30 minutes until the lentils are cooked through and you have a nice velvety Dahl.

Add the kale and coconut milk and cook another 5 minutes.

In the meantime, cook the buckwheat according to the package instructions with 1 teaspoon of turmeric, drain and serve along with the Dahl.

Baked tofu with harissa

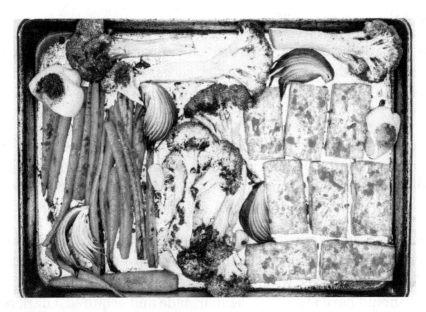

Ingredients for 1 persons:

- 60g of red bell pepper
- 1 Bird's Eye hot pepper
- 2 garlic cloves
- about 1 tablespoon of extra virgin olive oil
- 1 pinch of dried cumin
- 1 pinch of dried coriander
- juice of 1/4 lemon
- 200g of hard tofu
- 200g cauliflower, coarsely chopped
- 40g red onion, finely chopped
- 1 teaspoon fresh ginger, finely chopped
- 2 teaspoons turmeric powder
- 30g dried tomatoes, finely chopped
- 20g of chopped parsley

Preparation:

Heat the oven to 200°C.

To prepare the harissa, slice the bell pepper by turning it around the stem so that you get nice flat slices, remove the seeds and place the slices in a baking dish with the chili and one of the garlic cloves.

Season with a little oil and the dry spices and bake for 15-20 minutes until the bell pepper is soft but not too dark. (Leave the oven on at the same temperature.) Let cool, then blend in a food processor with the lemon juice until smooth.

Slice the tofu lengthwise and cut each slice into triangles. Place them in a small non-stick baking dish or covered with a sheet of baking paper, cover with harissa and bake for 20 minutes. The tofu should have absorbed the marinade and acquired a dark red color.

To prepare the "couscous," transfer the raw cauliflower to a food processor. Blend in short 2-second pulses until you get a couscous-like consistency. Or you can use a knife and chop it very finely.

Finely chop the remaining garlic clove. Sauté it with the red onion and ginger in 1 teaspoon of oil until wilted but not too brown, then add the turmeric and cauliflower and cook for 1 minute.

Remove from heat and add the sun-dried tomatoes and parsley. Serve with the baked tofu.

Paccheri in miso sauce, broccoli and dried apricots

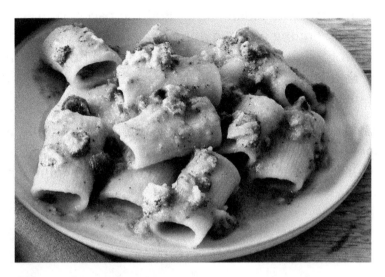

Ingredients for 4 persons:

- 320 g paccheri pasta
- 70 g broccoli florets
- 50 g anchovy fillets in oil
- 40 g miso (fermented soy-based condiment)
- 4 dried apricots
- 2 onions
- grated parmesan cheese
- extra virgin olive oil
- salt

Preparation:

For the recipe of paccheri in miso sauce, broccoli and dried apricots, slice the onions and stew them in a pan with 2 tablespoons of oil, on low heat, with the lid for 15-20 ': if necessary, add a ladle of hot water during cooking. Add the anchovies and continue for 10'. Remove the lid, reduce for 1 minute, add the miso, then blend until you have a sauce.

Cut the apricots into small cubes. Boil the paccheri in plenty of lightly salted boiling water, 5 minutes before the end of cooking add the broccoli florets and cook the pasta and florets. Drain the pasta with the broccoli and collect everything in the pan with the miso sauce.

Add the diced apricots and toss everything for 1 minute with 2 tablespoons of oil and 2 tablespoons of grana cheese. Season to taste with a grind of pepper and serve immediately piping hot.

Red quinoa salad

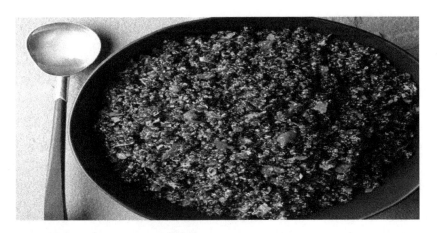

Ingredients for 6 persons:

FOR THE DRESSING

- 5 tablespoons of lime juice
- Salt 1 level teaspoon
- Garlic 1 clove
- Fresh coriander 50 g chopped
- Cumin 1 teaspoon
- Extra virgin olive oil 80 ml
- Pepper

FOR THE SALAD

- Quinoa 300 g
- Salt 1 tablespoon
- Black beans 250 g
- Peppers 150 g
- Chillies 1 chopped
- Chopped fresh coriander 50 g
- Chopped spring onions 100 g
- Corn 50 g boiled grains

Preparation:

In a bowl whisk together the lime juice, salt, minced garlic, chopped cilantro and cumin and add the oil while stirring. Add pepper to taste.

In a large bowl, wash the quinoa by changing the cold water at least 5 times, rubbing the grains and letting them settle to the bottom of the bowl before discarding the water; repeat this manoeuvre until the water is clean.

In a medium-sized pot, add the coarse salt and about 2 quarts of boiling water and boil the quinoa for 10 minutes. When finished cooking, drain the quinoa using a clean cloth as a strainer.

Pour the quinoa into a tureen, add the beans and all the vegetables chopped into small cubes, stir a little before adding the dressing, stir again and serve at room temperature.

Quinoa and tuna salad

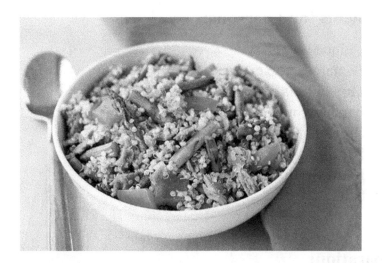

We offer you a healthy recipe of quinoa and tuna salad, easy and fast, perfect for those who suffer from celiac disease because quinoa, a vegetable that originates from a herbaceous plant which fruits in a panicle containing small seeds, does not have gluten. It is often confused for its appearance with cereals and, like cereals, it contains concentrations of starch, proteins, fibres, minerals and vitamins. This is one of the recipes for quinoa salads that you can then prepare as a first course or main course because, in addition to quinoa and tuna, includes tomatoes, parsley and green pepper, to make it a little 'special, spicy and fresh, as we will season it with lime juice, ideal for summer, also because it is light and low-calorie. If you don't like the taste of lime because it is too sour, you could add turmeric and make it spicier. How to cook quinoa is a frequent question, especially if you are not very familiar with ethnic dishes. The portion of raw quinoa grows about two and a half times, so you can assess how much you want to cook, we have considered a portion of 50 grams per person, but it also depends on the amount of other ingredients that will accompany it in the dish.

Ingredients for 4 persons:

- Quinoa 200 gr
- Tomatoes 300 gr
- Tinned tuna 250 gr
- Parsley 1 bunch
- Green pepper
- Lime juice 1
- Extra virgin olive oil two tablespoons
- Salt

Preparation:

Cooking quinoa is a simple and fast procedure, first of all you must soak the seeds for about half an hour in cold water, drain them and rinse them well in order to eliminate the saponin which covers them, and which gives quinoa a bitter taste in the mouth if not washed well.

In the meantime, put plenty of water in a pot and bring it to a boil.

Salt only while boiling, and then add the quinoa, let it cook for about 20 minutes. However, check the cooking time, which is complete when the seeds begin to become soft and transparent.

While the quinoa is cooking, prepare the other ingredients, wash the parsley and coarsely chop it.

When cooked, drain the quinoa and it will be ready to be simply seasoned.

Wash the tomatoes and cut them into pieces. A diced tomato made with a brunoised cut would be the most suitable for this operation, but if you can't do it, it's fine if you cut them into small pieces of roughly the same size.

Drain the excess oil from the tuna or use the natural tuna and break it up with a fork, leaving some larger pieces.

When the quinoa has cooled, place it in a large salad bowl, add the tomatoes and tuna and toss to combine.

Cut and squeeze some lime, then drizzle the salad with its juice and oil, salt and mix again.

Whole wheat penne with broccoli

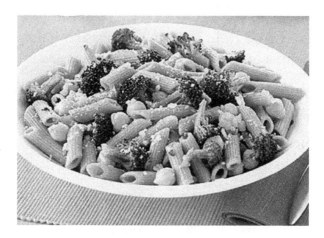

Ingredients for 4 persons:

- 280 g whole wheat penne
- 200 g broccoli florets
- 160 g parmesan cheese
- 80 g extra virgin olive oil
- 80 g onion
- Salt pepper

Preparation:

For the whole wheat penne with broccoli recipe, bring the water for the pasta to a boil, salt it and pour in the penne. Chop the onion and brown it gently in the oil for 5′; season with salt and pepper. Five minutes before the pasta is done cooking, add the broccoli florets, each divided into four. Finish cooking the pasta with the broccoli, drain and toss with the onion oil. Serve with plenty of grated cheese.

Quinoa with zucchini and pine nuts

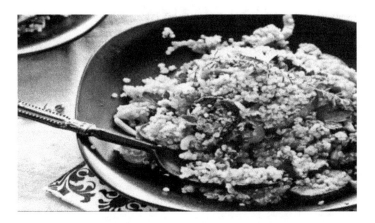

Ingredients for 4 persons:

- 150 gr of quinoa
- 2 of zucchini
- 1/2 of onion
- 20 gr of pine nuts
- mint
- salt
- olive oil

Preparation:

Rinse the quinoa well under running water to remove all traces of the bitter saponins.

Then place it in a pot with water: for each cup of quinoa you will need to add 2 cups of water.

Cook for 15 minutes from boiling.

In the meantime, cut the washed and trimmed zucchini into chunks.

Patricia Monroe

Chop the onion and fry it in a pan with a little oil.

Add the zucchini and let it brown in the pan before adding salt.

Add the pine nuts and mint and cook for a few more minutes.

Turn off the flame, add the quinoa and a drizzle of oil and stir.

Oriental prawns with buckwheat

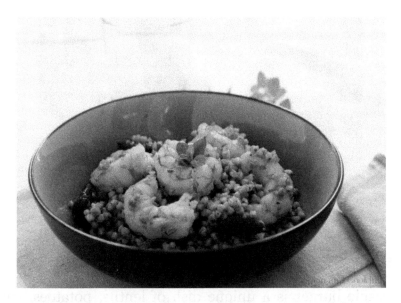

Cook 150 g shelled prawns in 1 teaspoon tamari and 1 teaspoon extra virgin olive oil for 2-3 minutes.

Boil 75 g of buckwheat noodles in unsalted water, drain and set aside.

Sauté with another teaspoon of extra virgin olive oil, 1 clove of garlic, 1 Bird's Eye chili pepper and 1 teaspoon of fresh ginger finely chopped, 20 g of red onion and 40 g of celery sliced, stir-fry.

40 g celery sliced, 75 g green beans chopped, 50 g kale coarsely chopped.

Add 100 ml of stock and bring to the boil, simmering until the vegetables are still crispy on the inside.

Add prawns, spaghetti and 5 g celery leaves, bring back to the boil and serve.

Veggie Burgers

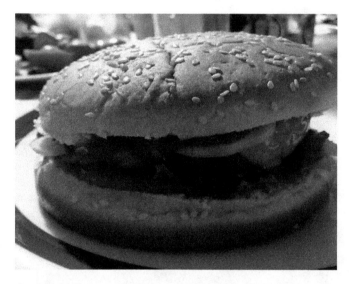

The veggie burger is a unique dish of lentils, potatoes, spring onions and herbs, which replaces meat burgers in the vegetarian diet. Brown the spring onion in oil, add the lentils, cover with water, add the herbs and bring to the boil. Then add the potatoes cut into pieces and cook for about 45 minutes. When the water has evaporated, mix the ingredients in a bowl and make your vegan burgers. Grease the burgers with evo oil and cook them in a pan for about 3 minutes per side. Once they are ready, you can dress them with a delicious pepper sauce or choose the seasoning and sauces you prefer according to your personal taste.

Eggplant burgers

Eggplant burgers are an easy second course to make: a vegetarian recipe that everyone will love, moreover it is prepared in a few minutes and allows you to use, among other things, stale bread. To prepare these vegetarian burgers it takes just a few steps: the aubergines are cut into pieces and cooked in a pan with a drizzle of oil, they are then added to bread softened with water, parmesan cheese and basil. Once ready you can serve your eggplant burgers with a tomato salad or mixed.

Chickpea burger

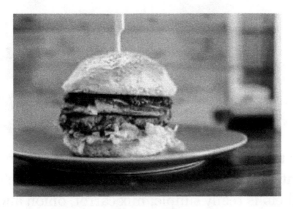

Chickpeas burgers are another delicious vegetarian and light version of the classic hamburger. Perfect even for those who have not chosen a diet free of meat and fish, they are a tasty alternative for enjoying chickpeas. The burgers are prepared by blending chickpeas with a few ingredients: egg, shallot, breadcrumbs and mustard. Once the ingredients are mixed together and the burgers are formed, pass them through breadcrumbs or cornmeal so that even those who cannot take gluten can enjoy them. Bake them in the oven for about 8 minutes per side and serve. Bring to the table some excellent chickpeas burgers, which you can enjoy by preparing a classic sandwich or if you prefer to accompany them with vegetables.

Lentil burger

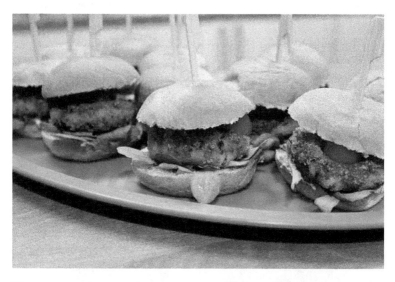

Lentil burgers are another Veggie variant of classic meat burger: they are light, tasty and very nutritious, as they are rich in protein. Preparing them is really simple: mix carrot, onion and parsley in the mixer. Then put the vegetables in a pan with the evo oil, drain the lentils previously put in water, and add them to the pot. Cover with water or vegetable stock and leave to cook for about 30 minutes. Blend everything together and form your vegetable hamburgers. Cook in a pan with a drizzle of oil and serve in a sandwich or with a fresh salad.

Chapter 7- Gluten-free

Braised beef with balsamic vinegar and onions

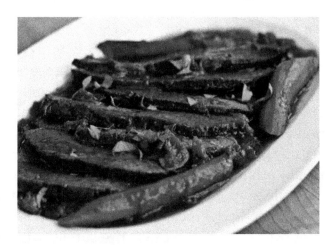

Ingredients for 4 persons:

- 1 kilo of beef priest's hat
- 300 grams of spring onions
- 2 carrots
- 2 celery ribs
- 150 milliliters of balsamic vinegar
- 200 millilitres of Barolo wine
- 5 cloves
- 1 cinnamon stick
- 1 handful of allspice
- 1 handful of black pepper
- 1 handful of rosemary
- 1 clove of garlic
- 1 teaspoon of juniper berries
- 4 leaves of sage
- enough extra virgin olive oil
- 2 tablespoons of worchestershire sause

- 1 handful of thyme

Preparation:

1. A main and important part which characterizes all braised meat recipes is the marinating usually done in wine, in this recipe we will make a dry marinating. Prepare in a food processor a generous handful of rosemary and sage along with berries such as allspice, black pepper and juniper, season with cloves and fresh garlic. Chop until you obtain a very fine powder in which all the herbs will be well mixed then add a pinch of salt and transfer the powder into a bowl in which you will also pour 2 tablespoons of balsamic vinegar of Modena. Place the piece of beef priest's hat on a cutting board and brush the entire surface with the spice mix, wrap it in plastic wrap and leave it to rest for at least twelve hours.
2. After the marinating and resting time of the meat we move on to the preparation of the dish. In a saucepan pour the Barolo wine and the balsamic vinegar of Modena together with the cinnamon stick, place over low heat and simmer until the mixture is reduced by fifty percent, then turn off the heat. In a frying pan pour a few tablespoons of extra virgin olive oil and brown, over high heat, the meat until it is well sealed. When golden brown, add the herbs, starting with the thyme, carrots and celery, then add the whole onions and 4 tablespoons of Worcestershire sauce. Sprinkle a pinch of salt over the vegetables and cover letting the meat cook for a few more minutes.
3. Add the reduction of Barolo, balsamic vinegar of Modena and cinnamon to the meat, cover again and bring to a boil, at this point lower the heat and cook the meat for about 3 hours. The last twenty minutes remove the lid and let the

liquid part shrink slightly. Once ready, let it cool and then slice it.

4. In a blender pour the cooking juices together with some onions, celery and carrots, removing the cinnamon, then blend until you have a light and creamy puree. Serve your braised meat with the onions and the blended cooking juices.

Baked high omelette

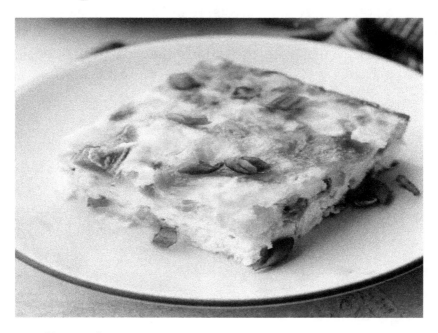

Ingredients for 4 persons:

- 4 eggs
- 250 grams of crescenza cheese
- 1 handful of parsley
- 1 handful of chives
- 1 pinch of black pepper
- 1 pinch of salt
- 3 tablespoons of parmesan cheese
- 1 tablespoon pecorino cheese
- 50 milliliters of whole milk

Preparation:

1. In a large bowl pour the whole eggs to which you will add the whole milk at room temperature, now with the help of a whisk beat vigorously the ingredients until you get a mixture airy and swollen. Add to the eggs a generous grinding of black pepper and a pinch of salt, and the parsley and chives finely chopped with a knife.

2. Continue preparing the omelette by adding the grated parmesan and pecorino cheese to the mixture and continue working vigorously with a whisk until all the ingredients are well blended together. Now prepare a baking pan for four portions and pour about three parts of the mixture into the bottom of the pan.

3. Place the crescenza cheese cut into pieces on top of the eggs and cover the entire surface; finish with the remaining egg mixture and bake in a preheated static oven at 180 degrees for about fifteen minutes. Once ready, remove from the oven and serve immediately.

Mullet fillets with aromatic herbs

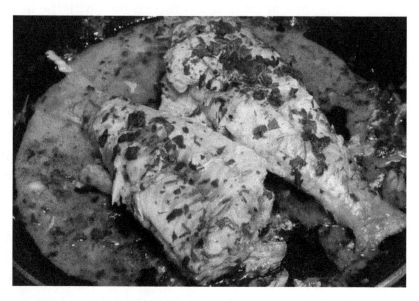

Ingredients for 2 persons:

- 350 grams of red mullet fillets
- 1 handful of pink pepper
- 1 handful of dill
- 4 sage leaves
- 1 clove of garlic
- 1 handful of parsley
- 1 handful of rosemary
- Enough fresh thyme
- enough butter
- 1 pinch of salt

Preparation:

1. On a cutting board place all the well washed and dried aromatic herbs and chop some such as parsley, dill and fresh thyme. Chop them finely in order to mix well all

98

the herbs. Set aside the sage leaves, rosemary and garlic clove. Prepare the herbs, then make the foil by placing a large sheet of baking paper on a flat surface. Sprinkle one half of the sheet of baking paper with half of the chopped herbs and half of the sage and rosemary. Lay the cleaned and boned red mullet fillets on the bed of herbs.

2. Cover the remaining fillets with the leftover herbs and chopped mixture, sprinkle with a pinch of salt and then add the crushed and coarsely chopped garlic clove. Finish with the pink peppercorns.

3. Add on the surface of the fillets a few knobs of butter and then go to close the wrapper of parchment paper and lay it on a baking sheet and heat the oven at a temperature of 200 degrees then cook the fillets for about 20 minutes. Once ready, remove the fish from the oven and serve immediately while still hot with all its aromas and seasonings.

Pan-fried broccoli

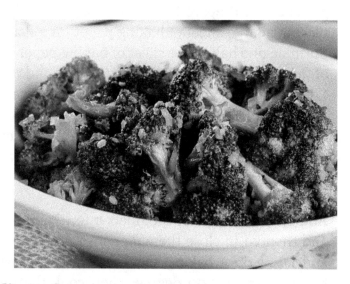

Ingredients for 4 persons:

- 2 broccoli
- 2 blond onions
- 50 grams of dried tomatoes
- 2 spoons of black olives in brine
- 2 tablespoons of Taggiasca olives
- 1 handful of fresh thyme
- sunflower seed oil
- salt

Preparation:

1. Clean the broccoli from the stem and the tougher leaves then divide all the florets and soak them in cold water for a few minutes, so that they can release all the impurities. Rinse the broccoli under plenty of cold water and boil it in salted water for a few minutes, until the stem is cooked but still crunchy. Drain the broccoli and stop the cooking

process by running it under a jet of cold water and set it aside.

2. Cover the bottom of a saucepan with a generous amount of sunflower oil and let it heat over a low flame. In the meantime, remove the outer leaves from the blond onions, cut them in half and slice them not too thinly, then pour them into the hot oil and add a pinch of salt. Cover and cook over low heat so that they do not burn. Let them cook until they become soft, almost transparent. On a chopping board, cut the sun-dried tomatoes into strips and a handful of black olives in brine into rounds; also prepare two tablespoons of olives that will enhance the flavor of the dish. When the onion is cooked and soft, add these last ingredients and let them continue to cook together over low heat so that the onion takes on the other flavors.

3. Scent with fresh thyme and add the previously boiled broccoli; mix all the ingredients together and put the lid back on then continue cooking until the broccoli is fully cooked. Turn off the flame and serve your broccoli while still hot.

Herb soup with chickpeas and speck

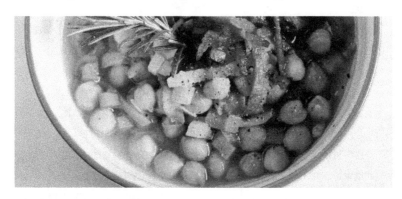

Ingredients for 2 persons:

- 400 grams of herbs
- 150 grams of speck
- 4 spring onions
- 150 grams of cooked chickpeas
- 1 tablespoon of sunflower oil
- enough salt
- 1 crust of grana padano cheese

Preparation:

1. Remove the outer skin from the fresh spring onions and cut them into coarse pieces; then do the same with the speck, after removing the rind, cut it into rather large cubes so as to preserve its flavor. In a large saucepan, toast the speck with a tablespoon of sunflower oil and when it becomes crispy, add the spring onions. Keeping the flame low, let them soften and brown without burning.
2. Wash the herbs thoroughly and several times in plenty of cold water to remove any residual soil. Cut them into pieces of the same size and add them to the fried bacon and

onion in the pot, raise the heat slightly and let them wilt slowly. When the herbs have reduced their volume, pour in the water that you have warmed up and cover them no more than two tablespoons above. Add just a pinch of salt and bring to a boil and at this point you can also add the crusts of grana Padano cheese in pieces well cleaned and netted. Cover with the lid and lower the heat, allowing the soup to cook for about twenty minutes.

3. After the first twenty minutes of cooking, remove the lid and add the cooked chickpeas, then cook for another fifteen minutes, after which turn off the heat. Let the soup cool down a little before serving it with some croutons.

Basmati rice with chicken and vegetables

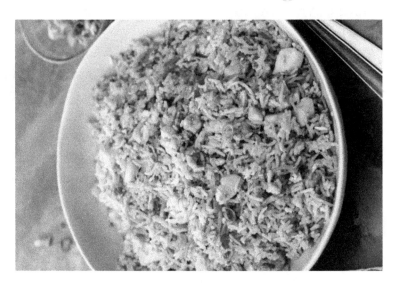

Ingredients for 4 persons:

- 500 grams of Chicken Breast
- 200 grams of Basmati Rice
- 2 Carrots
- 2 Courgettes
- 1 Onion
- 1 glass of White Wine
- 1 tablespoon of Turmeric
- Extra virgin olive oil
- Salt

Preparation:

1. To prepare basmati rice with chicken and vegetables, first wash the chicken breast and cut it into cubes. Put it in a pan with extra virgin olive oil, add salt, white wine and

turmeric. Cook it for 20 minutes. In another pan, sauté the sliced onion with the extra virgin olive oil.

2. Peel the carrots and cut them into thin strips using a potato peeler, then place them in the pan with the onion, add the soy sauce and cook for 10 minutes. Wash the zucchini, remove the ends and cut them with the potato peeler.

3. Add them to the pan, add salt and cook everything another 10 minutes. Then you will need to prepare the basmati rice. Boil some salted water in a saucepan, cook the rice in it for about 10 minutes then drain it and add some extra virgin olive oil.

Ligurian style meatloaf

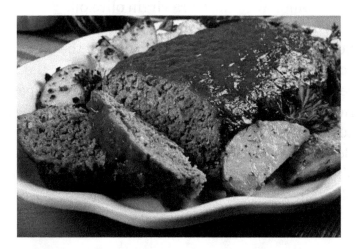

Ingredients for 6 persons:

- 600 grams of Potatoes
- 300 grams of Green Beans
- 50 grams of Parmesan
- 2 Eggs
- Nutmeg
- Extra Virgin Olive Oil
- Black Pepper
- Salt

Preparation:

1. To prepare the Ligurian-style meatloaf, first peel the potatoes, wash them and cut them into small pieces. Boil 2 litres of water in a saucepan and, when it boils, pour them in together with the green beans to which you have previously trimmed the ends. Cook for 20 minutes.

2. Once cooked, drain the vegetables, place them in a bowl and add salt. With an immersion blender, chop the mixture well, add the nutmeg, black pepper and Parmesan cheese.
3. After mixing, add the eggs and mix everything together. Grease an oven dish with extra virgin olive oil and pour in the meatloaf.
4. After 20 minutes of cooking in the oven at 180 degrees, the meatloaf is ready.

Patricia Monroe

APPENDIX

Cooking Conversion Charts

Volume (liquid)	
US Customary	Metric
1/8 teaspoon	0,6 ml
1/4 teaspoon	1.2 ml
1/2 teaspoon	2.5 ml
3/4 teaspoon	3.7 ml
1 teaspoon	5 ml
1 tablespoon	15 ml
2 tablespoon or 1 fluid ounce	30 ml
1/4 cup or 2 fluid ounces	59 ml
1/3 cup	79 ml
1/2 cup	118 ml
2/3 cup	158 ml
3/4 cup	177 ml
1 cup or 8 fluid ounces	237 ml
2 cups or 1 pint	473 ml
4 cups or 1 quart	946 ml
8 cups or 1/2 gallon	1.9 litres
1 gallon	3.8 litres

Weight (mass)	
US contemporary (ounces)	Metric (grams)
1/2 ounce	14 grams
1 ounce	28 grams
3 ounces	85 grams
3.53 ounces	100 grams
4 ounces	113 grams
8 ounces	227 grams
12 ounces	340 grams
16 ounces or 1 pound	454 grams

Oven Temperatures	
US contemporary	Metric
250° F	121° C
300° F	149° C
350° F	177° C
400° F	204° C
450° F	232° C

Volume Equivalents (liquid)		
3 teaspoons	1 tablespoon	0.5 fluid ounce
2 tablespoons	1/8 cup	1 fluid ounce
4 tablespoons	1/4 cup	2 fluid ounces
5 1/3 tablespoons	1/3 cup	2.7 fluid ounces
8 tablespoons	1/2 cup	4 fluid ounces
12 tablespoons	3/4 cup	6 fluid ounces
16 tablespoons	1 cup	8 fluid ounces
2 cups	1 pint	16 fluid ounces
2 pints	1 quart	32 fluid ounces
4 quarts	1 gallon	128 fluid ounces

CPSIA information can be obtained
at www.ICGtesting.com
Printed in the USA
LVHW020551290321
682791LV00005B/320

9 781802 354478